EASY KETO DIET RECIPES 2021

TASTY KETO RECIPES TO SURPRISE YOUR FRIENDS

SAMANTHA GREENE

Table of Contents

Introduction

Do you want to make a change in your life? Do you want to become a healthier person who can enjoy a new and improved life? Then, you are definitely in the right place. You are about to discover a wonderful and very healthy diet that has changed millions of lives. We are talking about the Ketogenic diet, a lifestyle that will mesmerize you and that will make you a new person in no time. So, let's sit back, relax and find out more about the Ketogenic diet.

A keto diet is a low carb one. This is the first and one of the most important things you should now. During such a diet, your body makes ketones in your liver and these are used as energy.
Your body will produce less insulin and glucose and a state of ketosis is induced.
Ketosis is a natural process that appears when our food intake is lower than usual. The body will soon adapt to this state and therefore you will be able to lose weight in no time but you will also become healthier and your physical and mental performances will improve.
Your blood sugar levels will improve and you won't be predisposed to diabetes.

Also, epilepsy and heart diseases can be prevented if you are on a Ketogenic diet.

Your cholesterol will improve and you will feel amazing in no time. How does that sound?

A Ketogenic diet is simple and easy to follow as long as you follow some simple rules. You don't need to make huge changes but there are some things you should know.

So, here goes!

Now let's start our magical culinary journey!

Ketogenic lifestyle...here we come!

Enjoy!

Juicy Pork Chops

These will be so tender and delicious!

Preparation time: 10 minutes

Cooking time: 45 minutes

Servings: 4

Ingredients:

- 2 yellow onions, chopped
- 6 bacon slices, chopped
- ½ cup chicken stock
- Salt and black pepper to the taste
- 4 pork chops

Directions:

1. Heat up a pan over medium heat, add bacon, stir, cook until it's crispy and transfer to a bowl.
2. Return pan to medium heat, add onions, some salt and pepper, stir, cover, cook for 15 minutes and transfer to the same bowl with the bacon.
3. Return pan once again to heat, increase to medium high, add pork chops, season with salt and pepper,

brown for 3 minutes on one side, flip, reduce heat to medium and cook for 7 minutes more.

4. Add stock, stir and cook for 2 minutes more.

5. Return bacon and onions to the pan, stir, cook for 1 minute more, divide between plates and serve.

Enjoy!

Nutrition: calories 325, fat 18, fiber 1, carbs 6, protein 36

Simple And Fast Pork Chops

This is going to be ready so fast!!

Preparation time: 10 minutes

Cooking time: 15 minutes

Servings: 4

Ingredients:

- 4 medium pork loin chops
- 1 teaspoon Dijon mustard
- 1 tablespoon Worcestershire sauce
- 1 teaspoon lemon juice
- 1 tablespoon water
- Salt and black pepper to the taste
- 1 teaspoon lemon pepper
- 1 tablespoon ghee
- 1 tablespoon chives, chopped

Directions:

1. In a bowl, mix water with Worcestershire sauce, mustard and lemon juice and whisk well.
2. Heat up a pan with the ghee over medium heat, add pork chops, season with salt, pepper and lemon pepper,

11

cook them for 6 minutes, flip and cook for 6 more minutes.

3. Transfer pork chops to a platter and keep them warm for now.
4. Heat up the pan again, pour mustard sauce you've made and bring to a gentle simmer.
5. Pour this over pork, sprinkle chives and serve.

Enjoy!

Nutrition: calories 132, fat 5, fiber 1, carbs 1, protein 18

Mediterranean Pork

This great keto dinner idea will make you feel great!

Preparation time: 10 minutes

Cooking time: 35 minutes

Servings: 4

Ingredients:

- 4 pork chops, bone-in
- Salt and black pepper to the taste
- 1 teaspoon rosemary, dried
- 3 garlic cloves, minced

Directions:

1. Season pork chops with salt and pepper and place in a roasting pan.
2. Add rosemary and garlic, introduce in the oven at 425 degrees F and bake for 10 minutes.
3. Reduce heat to 350 degrees F and roast for 25 minutes more.
4. Slice pork, divide between plates and drizzle pan juices all over.

Enjoy!

Nutrition: calories 165, fat 2, fiber 1, carbs 2, protein 26

Simple Pork Chops Delight

This is so yummy and simple to make at home!

Preparation time: 10 minutes

Cooking time: 40 minutes

Servings: 4

Ingredients:

- 4 pork chops
- 1 tablespoon oregano, chopped
- 2 garlic cloves, minced
- 1 tablespoon canola oil
- 15 ounces canned tomatoes, chopped
- 1 tablespoon tomato paste
- Salt and black pepper to the taste
- ¼ cup tomato juice

Directions:

1. Heat up a pan with the oil over medium high heat, add pork chops, season with salt and pepper, cook for 3 minutes, flip, cook for 3 minutes more and transfer to a plate.

2. Return pan to medium heat, add garlic, stir and cook for 10 seconds.
3. Add tomato juice, tomatoes and tomato paste, stir, bring to a boil and reduce heat to medium-low.
4. Add pork chops, stir, cover pan and simmer everything for 30 minutes.
5. Transfer pork chops to plates, add oregano to the pan, stir and cook for 2 minutes more.
6. Pour this over pork and serve.

Enjoy!

Nutrition: calories 210, fat 10, fiber 2, carbs 6, protein 19

Spicy Pork Chops

These spicy pork chops will impress you for sure!

Preparation time: 4 hours and 10 minutes

Cooking time: 15 minutes

Servings: 4

Ingredients:

- ¼ cup lime juice
- 4 pork rib chops
- 1 tablespoon coconut oil, melted
- 2 garlic cloves, minced
- 1 tablespoon chili powder
- 1 teaspoon cinnamon, ground
- 2 teaspoons cumin, ground
- Salt and black pepper to the taste
- ½ teaspoon hot pepper sauce
- Sliced mango for serving

Directions:

1. In a bowl, mix lime juice with oil, garlic, cumin, cinnamon, chili powder, salt, pepper and hot pepper sauce and whisk well.

17

2. Add pork chops, toss to coat and leave aside in the fridge for 4 hours.
3. Place pork on preheated grill over medium heat, cook for 7 minutes, flip and cook for 7 minutes more.
4. Divide between plates and serve with mango slices on the side.

Enjoy!

Nutrition: calories 200, fat 8, fiber 1, carbs 3, protein 26

Tasty Thai Beef

It will soon become your favorite keto dinner dish!

Preparation time: 10 minutes

Cooking time: 10 minutes

Servings: 6

Ingredients:

- 1 cup beef stock
- 4 tablespoons peanut butter
- ¼ teaspoon garlic powder
- ¼ teaspoon onion powder
- 1 tablespoon coconut aminos
- 1 and ½ teaspoons lemon pepper
- 1 pound beef steak, cut into strips
- Salt and black pepper to the taste
- 1 green bell pepper, chopped
- 3 green onions, chopped

Directions:

1. In a bowl, mix peanut butter with stock, aminos and lemon pepper, stir well and leave aside.

2. Heat up a pan over medium high heat, add beef, season with salt, pepper, onion and garlic powder and cook for 7 minutes.
3. Add green pepper, stir and cook for 3 minutes more.
4. Add peanut sauce you've made at the beginning and green onions, stir, cook for 1 minute more, divide between plates and serve.

Enjoy!

Nutrition: calories 224, fat 15, fiber 1, carbs 3, protein 19

The Best Beef Patties

This will be one of the best keto dishes you'll ever try!

Preparation time: 10 minutes

Cooking time: 35 minutes

Servings: 6

Ingredients:

- ½ cup bread crumbs
- 1 egg
- Salt and black pepper to the taste
- 1 and ½ pounds beef, ground
- 10 ounces canned onion soup
- 1 tablespoon coconut flour
- ¼ cup ketchup
- 3 teaspoons Worcestershire sauce
- ½ teaspoon mustard powder
- ¼ cup water

Directions:

1. In a bowl, mix 1/3 cup onion soup with beef, salt, pepper, egg and bread crumbs and stir well.

2. Heat up a pan over medium high heat, shape 6 patties from the beef mix, place them into the pan and brown on both sides.
3. Meanwhile, in a bowl, mix the rest of the soup with coconut flour, water, mustard powder, Worcestershire sauce and ketchup and stir well.
4. Pour this over beef patties, cover pan and cook for 20 minutes stirring from time to time.
5. Divide between plates and serve.

Enjoy!

Nutrition: calories 332, fat 18, fiber 1, carbs 7, protein 25

Amazing Beef Roast

It's so juicy and delicious!

Preparation time: 10 minutes

Cooking time: 1 hour and 15 minutes

Servings: 4

Ingredients:

- 3 and ½ pounds beef roast
- 4 ounces mushrooms, sliced
- 12 ounces beef stock
- 1 ounce onion soup mix
- ½ cup Italian dressing

Directions:

1. In a bowl, mix stock with onion soup mix and Italian dressing and stir.
2. Put beef roast in a pan, add mushrooms, stock mix, cover with tin foil, introduce in the oven at 300 degrees F and bake for 1 hour and 15 minutes.
3. Leave roast to cool down a bit, slice and serve with the gravy on top.

Enjoy!

Nutrition: calories 700, fat 56, fiber 2, carbs 10, protein 70

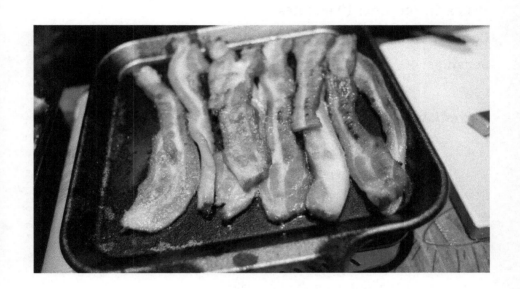

Beef Zucchini Cups

This looks so good and it tastes wonderful!

Preparation time: 10 minutes

Cooking time: 35 minutes

Servings: 4

Ingredients:

- 2 garlic cloves, minced
- 1 teaspoon cumin, ground
- 1 tablespoon coconut oil
- 1 pound beef, ground
- ½ cup red onion, chopped
- 1 teaspoon smoked paprika
- Salt and black pepper to the taste
- 3 zucchinis, sliced in halves lengthwise and insides scooped out
- ¼ cup cilantro, chopped
- ½ cup cheddar cheese, shredded
- 1 and ½ cups keto enchilada sauce
- Some chopped avocado for serving
- Some green onions, chopped for serving

- Some tomatoes, chopped for serving

Directions:

1. Heat up a pan with the oil over medium high heat, add red onions, stir and cook for 2 minutes.
2. Add beef, stir and brown for a couple of minutes.
3. Add paprika, salt, pepper, cumin and garlic, stir and cook for 2 minutes.
4. Place zucchini halves in a baking pan, stuff each with beef, pour enchilada sauce on top and sprinkle cheddar cheese.
5. Bake covered in the oven at 350 degrees F for 20 minutes.
6. Uncover the pan, sprinkle cilantro and bake for 5 minutes more.
7. Sprinkle avocado, green onions and tomatoes on top, divide between plates and serve.

Enjoy!

Nutrition: calories 222, fat 10, fiber 2, carbs 8, protein 21

Beef Meatballs Casserole

This is so special and of course, it's 100% keto!

Preparation time: 10 minutes

Cooking time: 50 minutes

Servings: 8

Ingredients:

- 1/3 cup almond flours
- 2 eggs
- 1 pound beef sausage, chopped
- 1 pound ground beef
- Salt and black pepper to taste
- 1 tablespoons parsley, dried
- ¼ teaspoon red pepper flakes
- ¼ cup parmesan, grated
- ¼ teaspoon onion powder
- ½ teaspoon garlic powder
- ¼ teaspoon oregano, dried
- 1 cup ricotta cheese
- 2 cups keto marinara sauce
- 1 and ½ cups mozzarella cheese, shredded

Directions:

1. In a bowl, mix sausage with beef, salt, pepper, almond flour, parsley, pepper flakes, onion powder, garlic powder, oregano, parmesan and eggs and stir well.
2. Shape meatballs, place them on a lined baking sheet, introduce in the oven at 375 degrees F and bake for 15 minutes.
3. Take meatballs out of the oven, transfer them to a baking dish and cover with half of the marinara sauce.
4. Add ricotta cheese all over, then pour the rest of the marinara sauce.
5. Sprinkle mozzarella all over, introduce dish in the oven at 375 degrees F and bake for 30 minutes.
6. Leave your meatballs casserole to cool down a bit before cutting and serving.

Enjoy!

Nutrition: calories 456, fat 35, fiber 3, carbs 4, protein 32

Beef And Tomato Stuffed Squash

It's always amazing to discover new and interesting dishes! This is one of them!

Preparation time: 10 minutes

Cooking time: 1 hour

Servings: 2

Ingredients:

- 2 pounds spaghetti squash, pricked with a fork
- Salt and black pepper to the taste
- 3 garlic cloves, minced
- 1 yellow onion, chopped
- 1 Portobello mushroom, sliced
- 28 ounces canned tomatoes, chopped
- 1 teaspoon oregano, dried
- ¼ teaspoon cayenne pepper
- ½ teaspoon thyme, dried
- 1 pound beef, ground
- 1 green bell pepper, chopped

Directions:

1. Place spaghetti squash on a lined baking sheet, introduce in the oven at 400 degrees F and bake for 40 minutes.
2. Cut in half, leave aside to cool down, remove seeds and leave aside.
3. Heat up a pan over medium high heat, add meat, garlic, onion and mushroom, stir and cook until meat browns.
4. Add salt, pepper, thyme, oregano, cayenne, tomatoes and green pepper, stir and cook for 10 minutes.
5. Stuff squash halves with this beef mix, introduce in the oven at 400 degrees F and bake for 10 minutes.
6. Divide between 2 plates and serve.

Enjoy!

Nutrition: calories 260, fat 7, fiber 2, carbs 4, protein 10

Tasty Beef Chili

This beef chili is so delightful! You've got to try this really soon!

Preparation time: 10 minutes

Cooking time: 8 hours

Servings: 4

Ingredients:

- 1 red onion, chopped
- 2 and ½ pounds beef, ground
- 15 ounces canned tomatoes and green chilies, chopped
- 6 ounces tomato paste
- ½ cup pickled jalapenos, chopped
- 4 tablespoons garlic, minced
- 3 celery ribs, chopped
- 2 tablespoons coconut aminos
- 4 tablespoons chili powder
- Salt and black pepper to the taste
- A pinch of cayenne pepper
- 2 tablespoons cumin, ground
- 1 teaspoon onion powder
- 1 teaspoon garlic powder

- 1 bay leaf
- 1 teaspoon oregano, dried

Directions:

1. Heat up a pan over medium high heat, add half of the onion, beef, half of the garlic, salt and pepper, stir and cook until meat browns.
2. Transfer this to your slow cooker, add the rest of the onion and garlic, but also, jalapenos, celery, tomatoes and chilies, tomato paste, canned tomatoes, coconut aminos, chili powder, salt, pepper, cumin, garlic powder, onion powder, oregano and bay leaf, stir, cover and cook on Low for 8 hours.
3. Divide into bowls and serve.

Enjoy!

Nutrition: calories 137, fat 6, fiber 2, carbs 5, protein 17

Glazed Beef Meatloaf

This will guarantee your success!

Preparation time: 10 minutes

Cooking time: 1 hour and 10 minutes

Servings: 6

Ingredients:

- 1 cup white mushrooms, chopped
- 3 pounds beef, ground
- 2 tablespoons parsley, chopped
- 2 garlic cloves, minced
- ½ cup yellow onion, chopped
- ¼ cup red bell pepper, chopped
- ½ cup almond flour
- 1/3 cup parmesan, grated
- 3 eggs
- Salt and black pepper to the taste
- 1 teaspoon balsamic vinegar
- *For the glaze:*
- 1 tablespoon swerve
- 2 tablespoons sugar-free ketchup

- 2 cups balsamic vinegar

Directions:

1. In a bowl, mix beef with salt, pepper, mushrooms, garlic, onion, bell pepper, parsley, almond flour, parmesan, 1 teaspoon vinegar, salt, pepper and eggs and stir very well.
2. Transfer this into a loaf pan and bake in the oven at 375 degrees F for 30 minutes.
3. Meanwhile, heat up a small pan over medium heat, add ketchup, swerve and 2 cups vinegar, stir well and cook for 20 minutes.
4. Take meatloaf out of the oven, spread the glaze over, introduce in the oven at the same temperature and bake for 20 minutes more.
5. Leave meatloaf to cool down, slice and serve it.

Enjoy!

Nutrition: calories 264, fat 14, fiber 3, carbs 5, protein 24

Delicious Beef And Tzatziki

You need to make sure there's enough for everyone!

Preparation time: 10 minutes

Cooking time: 15 minutes

Servings: 6

Ingredients:

- ¼ cup almond milk
- 17 ounces beef, ground
- 1 yellow onion, grated
- 5 bread slices, torn
- 1 egg, whisked
- ¼ cup parsley, chopped
- Salt and black pepper to the taste
- 2 garlic cloves, minced
- ¼ cup mint, chopped
- 2 and ½ teaspoons oregano, dried
- ¼ cup olive oil
- 7 ounces cherry tomatoes, cut in halves
- 1 cucumber, thinly sliced
- 1 cup baby spinach

- 1 and ½ tablespoons lemon juice
- 7 ounces jarred tzatziki

Directions:

1. Put torn bread in a bowl, add milk and leave aside for 3 minutes.
2. Squeeze bread, chop and put into a bowl.
3. Add beef, egg, salt, pepper, oregano, mint, parsley, garlic and onion and stir well.
4. Shape balls from this mix and place on a working surface.
5. Heat up a pan with half of the oil over medium high heat, add meatballs, cook them for 8 minutes flipping them from time to time and transfer them all to a tray.
6. In a salad bowl, mix spinach with cucumber and tomato.
7. Add meatballs, the rest of the oil, some salt, pepper and lemon juice.
8. Also add tzatziki, toss to coat and serve.

Enjoy!

Nutrition: calories 200, fat 4, fiber 1, carbs 3, protein 7

Meatballs And Tasty Mushroom Sauce

A friendly meal can turn into a feast with this keto dish!

Preparation time: 10 minutes

Cooking time: 25 minutes

Servings: 6

Ingredients:

- 2 pounds beef, ground
- Salt and black pepper to the taste
- ½ teaspoon garlic powder
- 1 tablespoon coconut aminos
- ¼ cup beef stock
- ¾ cup almond flour
- 1 tablespoon parsley, chopped
- 1 tablespoon onion flakes

For the sauce:

- 1 cup yellow onion, chopped
- 2 cups mushrooms, sliced
- 2 tablespoons bacon fat
- 2 tablespoons ghee
- ½ teaspoon coconut aminos

- ¼ cup sour cream
- ½ cup beef stock
- Salt and black pepper to the taste

Directions:

1. In a bowl, mix beef with salt, pepper, garlic powder, 1 tablespoons coconut aminos, ¼ cup beef stock, almond flour, parsley and onion flakes, stir well, shape 6 patties, place them on a baking sheet, introduce in the oven at 375 degrees F and bake for 18 minutes.
2. Meanwhile, heat up a pan with the ghee and the bacon fat over medium heat, add mushrooms, stir and cook for 4 minutes.
3. Add onions, stir and cook for 4 minutes more.
4. Add ½ teaspoon coconut aminos, sour cream and ½ cup beef stock, stir well and bring to a simmer.
5. Take off heat, add salt and pepper and stir well.
6. Divide beef patties between plates and serve with mushroom sauce on top.

Enjoy!

Nutrition: calories 435, fat 23, fiber 4, carbs 6, protein 32

Beef And Sauerkraut Soup

This beef and sauerkraut soup are so tasty!

Preparation time: 10 minutes

Cooking time: 1 hour and 20 minutes

Servings: 8

Ingredients:

- 3 teaspoons olive oil
- 1 pound beef, ground
- 14 ounces beef stock
- 2 cups chicken stock
- 14 ounces canned tomatoes and juice
- 1 tablespoon stevia
- 14 ounces sauerkraut, chopped
- 1 tablespoon gluten free Worcestershire sauce
- 4 bay leaves
- Salt and black pepper to the taste
- 3 tablespoons parsley, chopped
- 1 onion, chopped
- 1 teaspoon sage, dried
- 1 tablespoon garlic, minced

- 2 cups water

Directions:

1. Heat up a pan with 1 teaspoon oil over medium heat, add beef, stir and brown for 10 minutes.
2. Meanwhile, in a pot, mix chicken and beef stock with sauerkraut, stevia, canned tomatoes, Worcestershire sauce, parsley, sage and bay leaves, stir and bring to a simmer over medium heat.
3. Add beef to soup, stir and continue simmering.
4. Heat up the same pan with the rest of the oil over medium heat, add onions, stir and cook for 2 minutes. Add garlic, stir, cook for 1 minute more and add this to the soup.
5. Reduce heat to soup and simmer it for 1 hour.
6. Add salt, pepper and water, stir and cook for 15 minutes more.
7. Divide into bowls and serve.

Enjoy!

Nutrition: calories 250, fat 5, fiber 1, carbs 3, protein 12

Ground Beef Casserole

A friendly and casual meal requires such a keto dish!

Preparation time: 10 minutes

Cooking time: 35 minutes

Servings: 6

Ingredients:

- 2 teaspoons onion flakes
- 1 tablespoon gluten free Worcestershire sauce
- 2 pounds beef, ground
- 2 garlic cloves, minced
- Salt and black pepper to the taste
- 1 cup mozzarella cheese, shredded
- 2 cups cheddar cheese, shredded
- 1 cup Russian dressing
- 2 tablespoons sesame seeds, toasted
- 20 dill pickle slices
- 1 romaine lettuce head, torn

Directions:

1. Heat up a pan over medium heat, add beef, onion flakes, Worcestershire sauce, salt, pepper and garlic, stir and cook for 5 minutes.
2. Transfer this to a baking dish, add 1 cup cheddar cheese over it and also the mozzarella and half of the Russian dressing.
3. Stir and spread evenly.
4. Arrange pickle slices on top, sprinkle the rest of the cheddar and the sesame seeds, introduce in the oven at 350 degrees f and bake for 20 minutes.
5. Turn oven to broil and broil the casserole for 5 minutes more.
6. Divide lettuce on plates, top with a beef casserole and the rest of the Russian dressing.

Enjoy!

Nutrition: calories 554, fat 51, fiber 3, carbs 5, protein 45

Delicious Zoodles And Beef

It only takes a few minutes to make this special keto recipe!

Preparation time: 10 minutes

Cooking time: 20 minutes

Servings: 5

Ingredients:

- 1 pound beef, ground
- 1 yellow onion, chopped
- 2 garlic cloves, minced
- 14 ounces canned tomatoes, chopped
- 1 tablespoon rosemary, dried
- 1 tablespoon sage, dried
- 1 tablespoon oregano, dried
- 1 tablespoon basil, dried
- 1 tablespoon marjoram, dried
- Salt and black pepper to the taste
- 2 zucchinis, cut with a spiralizer

Directions:

1. Heat up a pan over medium heat, add garlic and onion, stir and brown for a couple of minutes.

2. Add beef, stir and cook for 6 minutes more.
3. Add tomatoes, salt, pepper, rosemary, sage, oregano, marjoram and basil, stir and simmer for 15 minutes.
4. Divide zoodles into bowls, add beef mix and serve.

Enjoy!

Nutrition: calories 320, fat 13, fiber 4, carbs 12, protein 40

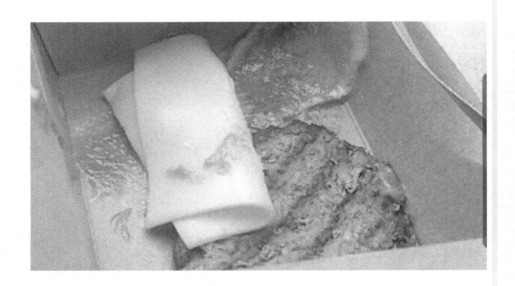

Jamaican Beef Pies

This is really tasty! You must make it for your family tonight!

Preparation time: 10 minutes

Cooking time: 35 minutes

Servings: 12

Ingredients:

- 3 garlic cloves, minced
- ½ pound beef, ground
- ½ pound pork, ground
- ½ cup water
- 1 small onion, chopped
- 2 habanero peppers, chopped
- 1 teaspoon Jamaican curry powder
- 1 teaspoon thyme, dried
- 2 teaspoons coriander, ground
- ½ teaspoon allspice
- 2 teaspoons cumin, ground
- ½ teaspoon turmeric
- A pinch of cloves, ground
- Salt and black pepper to the taste

- 1 teaspoon garlic powder
- ¼ teaspoon stevia powder
- 2 tablespoons ghee

For the crust:

- 4 tablespoons ghee, melted
- 6 ounces cream cheese
- A pinch of salt
- 1 teaspoon turmeric
- ¼ teaspoon stevia
- ½ teaspoon baking powder
- 1 and ½ cups flax meal
- 2 tablespoons water
- ½ cup coconut flour

Directions:

1. In your blender, mix onion with habaneros, garlic and ½ cup water.
2. Heat up a pan over medium heat, add pork and beef meat, stir and cook for 3 minutes.
3. Add onions mix, stir and cook for 2 minutes more.
4. Add garlic, onion, curry powder, ½ teaspoon turmeric, thyme, coriander, cumin, allspice, cloves, salt, pepper, stevia powder and garlic powder, stir well and cook for 3 minutes.
5. Add 2 tablespoons ghee, stir until it melts and take this off heat.
6. Meanwhile, in a bowl, mix 1 teaspoon turmeric, with ¼ teaspoon stevia, baking powder, flax meal and coconut flour and stir.
7. In a separate bowl, mix 4 tablespoons ghee with 2 tablespoons water and cream cheese and stir.
8. Combine the 2 mixtures and mix until you obtain a dough.
9. Shape 12 balls from this mix, place them on a parchment paper and roll each into a circle.
10. Divide beef and pork mix on one half of the dough circles, cover with the other halves, seal edges and arrange them all on a lined baking sheet.

11. Bake your pies in the oven at 350 degrees F for 25 minutes.
12. Serve them warm.

Enjoy!

Nutrition: calories 267, fat 23, fiber 1, carbs 3, protein 12

Amazing Goulash

This is a keto comfort food! Try it soon!

Preparation time: 10 minutes

Cooking time: 20 minutes

Servings: 5

Ingredients:

- 2 ounces bell pepper, chopped
- 1 and ½ pounds beef, ground
- Salt and black pepper to the taste
- 2 cups cauliflower florets
- ¼ cup onion, chopped
- 14 ounces canned tomatoes and their juice
- ¼ teaspoon garlic powder
- 1 tablespoon tomato paste
- 14 ounces water

Directions:

1. Heat up a pan over medium heat, add beef, stir and brown for 5 minutes.
2. Add onion and bell pepper, stir and cook for 4 minutes more.

3. Add cauliflower, tomatoes and their juice and water, stir, bring to a simmer, cover pan and cook for 5 minutes.
4. Add tomato paste, garlic powder, salt and pepper, stir, take off heat, divide into bowls and serve.

Enjoy!

Nutrition: calories 275, fat 7, fiber 2, carbs 4, protein 10

Beef And Eggplant Casserole

These ingredients go perfectly together!

Preparation time: 30 minutes

Cooking time: 4 hours

Servings: 12

Ingredients:

- 1 tablespoon olive oil
- 2 pounds beef, ground
- 2 cups eggplant, chopped
- Salt and black pepper to the taste
- 2 teaspoons mustard
- 2 teaspoons gluten free Worcestershire sauce
- 28 ounces canned tomatoes, chopped
- 2 cups mozzarella, grated
- 16 ounces tomato sauce
- 2 tablespoons parsley, chopped
- 1 teaspoon oregano, dried

Directions:

1. Season eggplant pieces with salt and pepper, leave them aside for 30 minutes, squeeze water a bit, put

53

them into a bowl, add the olive oil and toss them to coat.

2. In another bowl, mix beef with salt, pepper, mustard and Worcestershire sauce and stir well.
3. Press them on the bottom of a crock pot.
4. Add eggplant and spread.
5. Also add tomatoes, tomato sauce, parsley, oregano and mozzarella.
6. Cover Crockpot and cook on Low for 4 hours.
7. Divide casserole between plates and serve hot.

Enjoy!

Nutrition: calories 200, fat 12, fiber 2, carbs 6, protein 15

Braised Lamb Chops

It's a perfect keto dish!

Preparation time: 10 minutes

Cooking time: 2 hours and 20 minutes

Servings: 4

Ingredients:

- 8 lamb chops
- 1 teaspoon garlic powder
- Salt and black pepper to the taste
- 2 teaspoons mint, crushed
- A drizzle of olive oil
- 1 shallot, chopped
- 1 cup white wine
- Juice of ½ lemon
- 1 bay leaf
- 2 cups beef stock
- Some chopped parsley for serving

For the sauce:

- 2 cups cranberries
- ½ teaspoon rosemary, chopped
- ½ cup swerve
- 1 teaspoon mint, dried

- Juice of ½ lemon
- 1 teaspoon ginger, grated
- 1 cup water
- 1 teaspoon harissa paste

Directions:

1. In a bowl, mix lamb chops with salt, pepper, 1 teaspoon garlic powder and 2 teaspoons mint and rub well.
2. Heat up a pan with a drizzle of oil over medium high heat, add lamb chops, brown them on all sides and transfer to a plate.
3. Heat up the same pan again over medium high heat, add shallots, stir and cook for 1 minute.
4. Add wine and bay leaf, stir and cook for 4 minutes.
5. Add 2 cups beef stock, parsley and juice from ½ lemon, stir and simmer for 5 minutes.
6. Return lamb, stir and cook for 10 minutes.
7. Cover pan and introduce it in the oven at 350 degrees F for 2 hours.
8. Meanwhile, heat up a pan over medium high heat, add cranberries, swerve, rosemary, 1 teaspoon mint, juice from ½ lemon, ginger, water and harissa paste, stir, bring to a simmer for 15 minutes.
9. Take lamb chops out of the oven, divide them between plates, drizzle the cranberry sauce over them and serve.

Nutrition: calories 450, fat 34, fiber 2, carbs 6, protein 26

Amazing Lamb Salad

It's a flavored salad you should try in the summer!

Preparation time: 10 minutes

Cooking time: 35 minutes

Servings: 4

Ingredients:

- 1 tablespoon olive oil
- 3 pounds leg of lamb, bone discarded and butterflied
- Salt and black pepper to the taste
- 1 teaspoon cumin, ground
- A pinch of thyme, dried
- 2 garlic cloves, minced

For the salad:

- 4 ounces feta cheese, crumbled
- ½ cup pecans
- 2 cups spinach
- 1 and ½ tablespoons lemon juice
- ¼ cup olive oil
- 1 cup mint, chopped

Directions:

1. Rub lamb with salt, pepper, 1 tablespoon oil, thyme, cumin and minced garlic, place on preheated grill over medium high heat and cook for 40 minutes, flipping once.
2. Meanwhile, spread pecans on a lined baking sheet, introduce in the oven at 350 degrees F and toast for 10 minutes.
3. Transfer grilled lamb to a cutting board, leave aside to cool down and slice.
4. In a salad bowl, mix spinach with 1 cup mint, feta cheese, ¼ cup olive oil, lemon juice, toasted pecans, salt and pepper and toss to coat.
5. Add lamb slices on top and serve.

Enjoy!

Nutrition: calories 334, fat 33, fiber 3, carbs 5, protein 7

Moroccan Lamb

Try this Moroccan keto dish as soon as you can!

Preparation time: 10 minutes

Cooking time: 15 minutes

Servings: 4

Ingredients:

- 2 teaspoons paprika
- 2 garlic cloves, minced
- 2 teaspoons oregano, dried
- 2 tablespoons sumac
- 12 lamb cutlets
- ¼ cup olive oil
- 2 tablespoons water
- 2 teaspoons cumin, ground
- 4 carrots, sliced
- ¼ cup parsley, chopped
- 2 teaspoons harissa
- 1 tablespoon red wine vinegar
- Salt and black pepper to the taste
- 2 tablespoons black olives, pitted and sliced

- 6 radishes, thinly sliced

Directions:

1. In a bowl, mix cutlets with paprika, garlic, oregano, sumac, salt, pepper, half of the oil and the water and rub well.
2. Put carrots in a pot, add water to cover, bring to a boil over medium high heat, cook for 2 minutes drain and put them in a salad bowl.
3. Add olives and radishes over carrots.
4. In another bowl, mix harissa with the rest of the oil, parsley, cumin, vinegar and a splash of water and stir well.
5. Add this to carrots mix, season with salt and pepper and toss to coat.
6. Heat up a kitchen grill over medium high heat, add lamb cutlets, grill them for 3 minutes on each side and divide them between plates.
7. Add carrots salad on the side and serve.

Enjoy!

Nutrition: calories 245, fat 32, fiber 6, carbs 4, protein 34

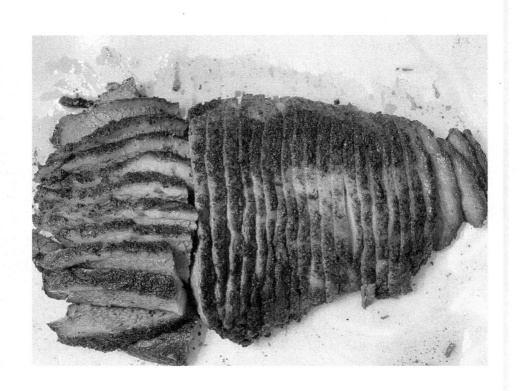

Delicious Lamb And Mustard Sauce

It's so rich and flavored and it's ready in only half an hour!

Preparation time: 10 minutes

Cooking time: 20 minutes

Servings: 4

Ingredients:

- 2 tablespoons olive oil
- 1 tablespoon fresh rosemary, chopped
- 2 garlic cloves, minced
- 1 and ½ pounds lamb chops
- Salt and black pepper to the taste
- 1 tablespoon shallot, chopped
- 2/3 cup heavy cream
- ½ cup beef stock
- 1 tablespoon mustard
- 2 teaspoons gluten free Worcestershire sauce
- 2 teaspoons lemon juice
- 1 teaspoon erythritol
- 2 tablespoons ghee
- A spring of rosemary

- A spring of thyme

Directions:

1. In a bowl, mix 1 tablespoon oil with garlic, salt, pepper and rosemary and whisk well.
2. Add lamb chops, toss to coat and leave aside for a few minutes.
3. Heat up a pan with the rest of the oil over medium high heat, add lamb chops, reduce heat to medium, cook them for 7 minutes, flip, cook them for 7 minutes more, transfer to a plate and keep them warm.
4. Return pan to medium heat, add shallots, stir and cook for 3 minutes.
5. Add stock, stir and cook for 1 minute.
6. Add Worcestershire sauce, mustard, erythritol, cream, rosemary and thyme spring, stir and cook for 8 minutes.
7. Add lemon juice, salt, pepper and the ghee, discard rosemary and thyme, stir well and take off heat.
8. Divide lamb chops on plates, drizzle the sauce over them and serve.

Enjoy!

Nutrition: calories 435, fat 30, fiber 4, carbs 5, protein 32

Tasty Lamb Curry

This lamb curry is going to surprise you for sure!

Preparation time: 10 minutes

Cooking time: 4 hours

Servings: 6

Ingredients:

- 2 tablespoons ginger, grated
- 2 garlic cloves, minced
- 2 teaspoons cardamom
- 1 red onion, chopped
- 6 cloves
- 1 pound lamb meat, cubed
- 2 teaspoons cumin powder
- 1 teaspoon garama masala
- ½ teaspoon chili powder
- 1 teaspoon turmeric
- 2 teaspoons coriander, ground
- 1 pound spinach
- 14 ounces canned tomatoes, chopped

Directions:

1. In your slow cooker, mix lamb with spinach, tomatoes, ginger, garlic, onion, cardamom, cloves, cumin, garam masala, chili, turmeric and coriander, stir, cover and cook on High for 4 hours.

2. Uncover slow cooker, stir your chili, divide into bowls and serve.

Enjoy!

Nutrition: calories 160, fat 6, fiber 3, carbs 7, protein 20

Tasty Lamb Stew

Don't bother looking for a Ketogenic dinner idea! This is the perfect one!

Preparation time: 10 minutes

Cooking time: 3 hours

Servings: 4

Ingredients:

- 1 yellow onion, chopped
- 3 carrots, chopped
- 2 pounds lamb, cubed
- 1 tomato, chopped
- 1 garlic clove, minced
- 2 tablespoons ghee
- 1 cup beef stock
- 1 cup white wine
- Salt and black pepper to the taste
- 2 rosemary springs
- 1 teaspoon thyme, chopped

Directions:

1. Heat up a Dutch oven over medium high heat, add oil and heat up.
2. Add lamb, salt and pepper, brown on all sides and transfer to a plate.
3. Add onion to the pot and cook for 2 minutes.
4. Add carrots, tomato, garlic, ghee, stick, wine, salt, pepper, rosemary and thyme, stir and cook for a couple of minutes.
5. Return lamb to pot, stir, reduce heat to medium low, cover and cook for 4 hours.
6. Discard rosemary springs, add more salt and pepper, stir, divide into bowls and serve.

Enjoy!

Nutrition: calories 700, fat 43, fiber 6, carbs 10, protein 67

Delicious Lamb Casserole

Serve this keto dish on a Sunday!

Preparation time: 10 minutes

Cooking time: 1 hour and 40 minutes

Servings: 2

Ingredients:

- 2 garlic cloves, minced
- 1 red onion, chopped
- 1 tablespoon olive oil
- 1 celery stick, chopped
- 10 ounces lamb fillet, cut into medium pieces
- Salt and black pepper to the taste
- 1 and ¼ cups lamb stock
- 2 carrots, chopped
- ½ tablespoon rosemary, chopped
- 1 leek, chopped
- 1 tablespoon mint sauce
- 1 teaspoon stevia
- 1 tablespoon tomato puree
- ½ cauliflower, florets separated

- ½ celeriac, chopped
- 2 tablespoons ghee

Directions:

1. Heat up a pot with the oil over medium heat, add garlic, onion and celery, stir and cook for 5 minutes.
2. Add lamb pieces, stir and cook for 3 minutes.
3. Add carrot, leek, rosemary, stock, tomato puree, mint sauce and stevia, stir, bring to a boil, cover and cook for 1 hour and 30 minutes.
4. Heat up a pot with water over medium heat, add celeriac, cover and simmer for 10 minutes.
5. Add cauliflower florets, cook for 15 minutes, drain everything and mix with salt, pepper and ghee.
6. Mash using a potato masher and divide mash between plates.
7. Add lamb and veggies mix on top and serve.

Enjoy!

Nutrition: calories 324, fat 4, fiber 5, carbs 8, protein 20

Cheesy Chicken

Your friends will ask for more!

Preparation time: 10 minutes

Cooking time: 30 minutes

Servings: 4

Ingredients:

- 1 zucchini, chopped
- Salt and black pepper to the taste
- 1 teaspoon garlic powder
- 1 tablespoon avocado oil
- 2 chicken breasts, skinless and boneless and sliced
- 1 tomato, chopped
- ½ teaspoon oregano, dried
- ½ teaspoon basil, dried
- ½ cup mozzarella cheese, shredded

Directions:

1. Season chicken with salt, pepper and garlic powder.
2. Heat up a pan with the oil over medium heat, add chicken slices, brown on all sides and transfer them to a baking dish.

3. Heat up the pan again over medium heat, add zucchini, oregano, tomato, basil, salt and pepper, stir, cook for 2 minutes and pour over chicken.
4. Introduce in the oven at 325 degrees F and bake for 20 minutes.
5. Spread mozzarella over chicken, introduce in the oven again and bake for 5 minutes more.
6. Divide between plates and serve.

Enjoy!

Nutrition: calories 235, fat 4, fiber 1, carbs 2, protein 35

Orange Chicken

The combination is absolutely delicious!

Preparation time: 10 minutes

Cooking time: 15 minutes

Servings: 4

Ingredients:

- 2 pounds chicken thighs, skinless, boneless and cut into pieces
- Salt and black pepper to the taste
- 3 tablespoons coconut oil
- ¼ cup coconut flour

For the sauce:

- 2 tablespoons fish sauce
- 1 and ½ teaspoons orange extract
- 1 tablespoon ginger, grated
- ¼ cup orange juice
- 2 teaspoons stevia
- 1 tablespoon orange zest
- ¼ teaspoon sesame seeds
- 2 tablespoons scallions, chopped

- ½ teaspoon coriander, ground
- 1 cup water
- ¼ teaspoon red pepper flakes
- 2 tablespoons gluten free soy sauce

Directions:

1. In a bowl, mix coconut flour and salt and pepper and stir.
2. Add chicken pieces and toss to coat well.
3. Heat up a pan with the oil over medium heat, add chicken, cook until they are golden on both sides and transfer to a bowl.
4. In your blender, mix orange juice with ginger, fish sauce, soy sauce, stevia, orange extract, water and coriander and blend well.
5. Pour this into a pan and heat up over medium heat.
6. Add chicken, stir and cook for 2 minutes.
7. Add sesame seeds, orange zest, scallions and pepper flakes, stir cook for 2 minutes and take off heat.
8. Divide between plates and serve.

Enjoy!

Nutrition: calories 423, fat 20, fiber 5, carbs 6, protein 45

Chicken Pie

This pie is so delicious!

Preparation time: 10 minutes

Cooking time: 45 minutes

Servings: 4

Ingredients:

- ½ cup yellow onion, chopped
- 3 tablespoons ghee
- ½ cup carrots, chopped
- 3 garlic cloves, minced
- Salt and black pepper to the taste
- ¾ cup heavy cream
- ½ cup chicken stock
- 12 ounces chicken, cubed
- 2 tablespoons Dijon mustard
- ¾ cup cheddar cheese, shredded

For the dough:

- ¾ cup almond flour
- 3 tablespoons cream cheese
- 1 and ½ cup mozzarella cheese, shredded
- 1 egg

- 1 teaspoon onion powder
- 1 teaspoon garlic powder
- 1 teaspoon Italian seasoning
- Salt and black pepper to the taste

Directions:

1. Heat up a pan with the ghee over medium heat, add onion, carrots, garlic, salt and pepper, stir and cook for 5 minutes.
2. Add chicken, stir and cook for 3 minutes more.
3. Add heavy cream, stock, salt, pepper and mustard, stir and cook for 7 minutes more.
4. Add cheddar cheese, stir well, take off heat and keep warm.
5. Meanwhile, in a bowl, mix mozzarella with cream cheese, stir and heat up in your microwave for 1 minute.
6. Add garlic powder, Italian seasoning, salt, pepper, onion powder, flour and egg and stir well.

7. Knead your dough very well, divide into 4 pieces and flatten each into a circle.
8. Divide chicken mix into 4 ramekins, top each with a dough circle, introduce in the oven at 375 degrees F for 25 minutes.
9. Serve your chicken pies warm.

Enjoy!

Nutrition: calories 600, fat 54, fiber 14, carbs 10, protein 45

Bacon Wrapped Chicken

The flavors will hypnotize you for sure!

Preparation time: 10 minutes

Cooking time: 35 minutes

Servings: 4

Ingredients:

- 1 tablespoon chives, chopped
- 8 ounces cream cheese
- 2 pounds chicken breasts, skinless and boneless
- 12 bacon slices
- Salt and black pepper to the taste

Directions:

1. Heat up a pan over medium heat, add bacon, cook until it's half done, transfer to paper towels and drain grease.
2. In a bowl, mix cream cheese with salt, pepper and chives and stir.
3. Use a meat tenderizer to flatten chicken breasts well, divide cream cheese mix, roll them up and wrap each in a cooked bacon slice.

4. Arrange wrapped chicken breasts into a baking dish, introduce in the oven at 375 degrees F and bake for 30 minutes.

5. Divide between plates and serve.

Enjoy!

Nutrition: calories 700, fat 45, fiber 4, carbs 5, protein 45

So Delicious Chicken Wings

You will fall in love with this keto dish and you will make it over and over again!

Preparation time: 10 minutes

Cooking time: 55 minutes

Servings: 4

Ingredients:

- 3 pounds chicken wings
- Salt and black pepper to the taste
- 3 tablespoons coconut aminos
- 2 teaspoons white vinegar
- 3 tablespoons rice vinegar
- 3 tablespoons stevia
- ¼ cup scallions, chopped
- ½ teaspoon xanthan gum
- 5 dried chilies, chopped

Directions:

1. Spread chicken wings on a lined baking sheet, season with salt and pepper, introduce in the oven at 375 degrees F and bake for 45 minutes.

2. Meanwhile, heat up a small pan over medium heat, add white vinegar, rice vinegar, coconut aminos, stevia, xanthan gum, scallions and chilies, stir well, bring to a boil, cook for 2 minutes and take off heat.
3. Dip chicken wings into this sauce, arrange them all on the baking sheet again and bake for 10 minutes more.
4. Serve them hot.

Enjoy!

Nutrition: calories 415, fat 23, fiber 3, carbs 2, protein 27

Chicken In Creamy Sauce

Trust us! This keto recipe is here to impress you!

Preparation time: 10 minutes

Cooking time: 1 hour and 10 minutes

Servings: 4

Ingredients:

- 8 chicken thighs
- Salt and black pepper to the taste
- 1 yellow onion, chopped
- 1 tablespoon coconut oil
- 4 bacon strips, chopped
- 4 garlic cloves, minced
- 10 ounces cremini mushrooms, halved
- 2 cups white chardonnay wine
- 1 cup whipping cream
- A handful parsley, chopped

Directions:

1. Heat up a pan with the oil over medium heat, add bacon, stir, cook until it's crispy, take off heat and transfer to paper towels.
2. Heat up the pan with the bacon fat over medium heat, add chicken pieces, season them with salt and pepper, cook until they brown and also transfer to paper towels.
3. Heat up the pan again over medium heat, add onions, stir and cook for 6 minutes.
4. Add garlic, stir, cook for 1 minute and transfer next to bacon pieces.
5. Return pan to stove and heat up again over medium temperature.
6. Add mushrooms stir and cook them for 5 minutes.
7. Return chicken, bacon, garlic and onion to pan.
8. Add wine, stir, bring to a boil, reduce heat and simmer for 40 minutes.
9. Add parsley and cream, stir and cook for 10 minutes more.
10. Divide between plates and serve.

Enjoy!

Nutrition: calories 340, fat 10, fiber 7, carbs 4, protein 24

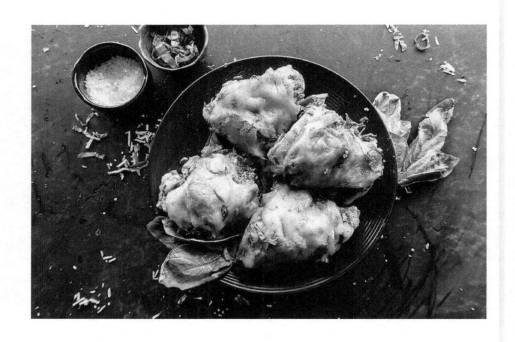

Delightful Chicken

It's a delicious and textured keto poultry dish!

Preparation time: 10 minutes

Cooking time: 1 hour

Servings: 4

Ingredients:

- 6 chicken breasts, skinless and boneless
- Salt and black pepper to the taste
- ¼ cup jalapenos, chopped
- 5 bacon slices, chopped
- 8 ounces cream cheese
- ¼ cup yellow onion, chopped
- ½ cup mayonnaise
- ½ cup parmesan, grated
- 1 cup cheddar cheese, grated

For the topping:

- 2 ounces pork skins, crushed
- 4 tablespoons melted ghee
- ½ cup parmesan

Directions:

1. Arrange chicken breasts in a baking dish, season with salt and pepper, introduce in the oven at 425 degrees F and bake for 40 minutes.
2. Meanwhile, heat up a pan over medium heat, add bacon, stir, cook until it's crispy and transfer to a plate.
3. Heat up the pan again over medium heat, add onions, stir and cook for 4 minutes.
4. Take off heat, add bacon, jalapeno, cream cheese, mayo, cheddar cheese and ½ cup parm and stir well..
5. Spread this over chicken.
6. In a bowl, mix pork skin with ghee and ½ cup parm and stir.
7. Spread this over chicken as well, introduce in the oven and bake for 15 minutes more.
8. Serve hot.

Enjoy!

Nutrition: calories 340, fat 12, fiber 2, carbs 5, protein 20

Tasty Chicken And Sour Cream Sauce

You've got to learn how to make this tasty keto dish! It's so tasty!

Preparation time: 10 minutes

Cooking time: 40 minutes

Servings: 4

Ingredients:

- 4 chicken thighs
- Salt and black pepper to the taste
- 1 teaspoon onion powder
- ¼ cup sour cream
- 2 tablespoons sweet paprika

Directions:

1. In a bowl, mix paprika with salt, pepper and onion powder and stir.
2. Season chicken pieces with this paprika mix, arrange them on a lined baking sheet and bake in the oven at 400 degrees F for 40 minutes.

3. Divide chicken on plates and leave aside for now.
4. Pour juices from the pan into a bowl and add sour cream.
5. Stir this sauce very well and drizzle over chicken.

Enjoy!

Nutrition: calories 384, fat 31, fiber 2, carbs 1, protein 33

Tasty Chicken Stroganoff

Have you heard about this keto recipe? It seems it's amazing!

Preparation time: 10 minutes

Cooking time: 4 hours and 10 minutes

Servings: 4

Ingredients:

- 2 garlic cloves, minced
- 8 ounces mushrooms, roughly chopped
- ¼ teaspoon celery seeds, ground
- 1 cup chicken stock
- 1 cup coconut milk
- 1 yellow onion, chopped
- 1 pound chicken breasts, cut into medium pieces
- 1 and ½ teaspoons thyme, dried
- 2 tablespoons parsley, chopped
- Salt and black pepper to the teste
- 4 zucchinis, cut with a spiralizer

Directions:

1. Put chicken in your slow cooker.

2. Add salt, pepper, onion, garlic, mushrooms, coconut milk, celery seeds, stock, half of the parsley and thyme.

3. Stir, cover and cook on High for 4 hours.

4. Uncover pot, add more salt and pepper if needed and the rest of the parsley and stir.

5. Heat up a pan with water over medium heat, add some salt, bring to a boil, add zucchini pasta, cook for 1 minute and drain.

6. Divide on plates, add chicken mix on top and serve.

Enjoy!

Nutrition: calories 364, fat 22, fiber 2, carbs 4, protein 24

Tasty Chicken Gumbo

Oh. You are going to love this!

Preparation time: 10 minutes

Cooking time: 7 hours

Servings: 5

Ingredients:

- 2 sausages, sliced
- 3 chicken breasts, cubed
- 2 tablespoons oregano, dried
- 2 bell peppers, chopped
- 1 small yellow onion, chopped
- 28 ounces canned tomatoes, chopped
- 3 tablespoons thyme, dried
- 2 tablespoons garlic powder
- 2 tablespoons mustard powder
- 1 teaspoon cayenne powder
- 1 tablespoons chili powder
- Salt and black pepper to the taste
- 6 tablespoons Creole seasoning

Directions:

1. In your slow cooker, mix sausages with chicken pieces, salt, pepper, bell peppers, oregano, onion, thyme, garlic powder, mustard powder, tomatoes, cayenne, chili and Creole seasoning.
2. Cover and cook on Low for 7 hours.
3. Uncover pot again, stir gumbo and divide into bowls.
4. Serve hot.

Enjoy!

Nutrition: calories 360, fat 23, fiber 2, carbs 6, protein 23

Tender Chicken Thighs

You'll see what we're talking about!

Preparation time: 10 minutes

Cooking time: 45 minutes

Servings: 4

Ingredients:

- 3 tablespoons ghee
- 8 ounces mushrooms, sliced
- 2 tablespoons gruyere cheese, grated
- Salt and black pepper to the taste
- 2 garlic cloves, minced
- 6 chicken thighs, skin and bone-in

Directions:

1. Heat up a pan with 1 tablespoon ghee over medium heat, add chicken thighs, season with salt and pepper, cook for 3 minutes on each side and arrange them in a baking dish.
2. Heat up the pan again with the rest of the ghee over medium heat, add garlic, stir and cook for 1 minute.
3. Add mushrooms and stir well.

4. Add salt and pepper, stir and cook for 10 minutes.
5. Spoon these over chicken, sprinkle cheese, introduce in the oven at 350 degrees F and bake for 30 minutes.
6. Turn oven to broiler and broil everything for a couple more minutes.
7. Divide between plates and serve.

Enjoy!

Nutrition: calories 340, fat 31, fiber 3, carbs 5, protein 64

Tasty Crusted Chicken

This is just perfect!

Preparation time: 10 minutes

Cooking time: 20 minutes

Servings: 4

Ingredients:

- 1 egg, whisked
- Salt and black pepper to the taste
- 3 tablespoons coconut oil
- 1 and ½ cups pecans, chopped
- 4 chicken breasts
- Salt and black pepper to the taste

Directions:

1. Put pecans in a bowl and the whisked egg in another.
2. Season chicken, dip in egg and then in pecans.
3. Heat up a pan with the oil over medium high heat, add chicken and cook until it's brown on both sides.
4. Transfer chicken pieces to a baking sheet, introduce in the oven and bake at 350 degrees F for 10 minutes.
5. Divide between plates and serve.

Enjoy!

Nutrition: calories 320, fat 12, fiber 4, carbs 1, protein 30

Pepperoni Chicken Bake

It's impossible not to appreciate this great keto dish!

Preparation time: 10 minutes

Cooking time: 55 minutes

Servings: 6

Ingredients:

- 14 ounces low carb pizza sauce
- 1 tablespoon coconut oil
- 4 medium chicken breasts, skinless and boneless
- Salt and black pepper to the taste
- 1 teaspoon oregano, dried
- 6 ounces mozzarella, sliced
- 1 teaspoon garlic powder
- 2 ounces pepperoni, sliced

Directions:

1. Put pizza sauce in a small pot, bring to a boil over medium heat, simmer for 20 minutes and take off heat.
2. In a bowl, mix chicken with salt, pepper, garlic powder and oregano and stir.

3. Heat up a pan with the coconut oil over medium high heat, add chicken pieces, cook for 2 minutes on each side and transfer them to a baking dish.
4. Add mozzarella slices on top, spread sauce, top with pepperoni slices, introduce in the oven at 400 degrees F and bake for 30 minutes.
5. Divide between plates and serve.

Enjoy!

Nutrition: calories 320, fat 10, fiber 6, carbs 3, protein 27

Fried Chicken

It's a very simple dish you will like!

Preparation time: 24 hours

Cooking time: 20 minutes

Servings: 4

Ingredients:

- 3 chicken breasts, cut into strips
- 4 ounces pork rinds, crushed
- 2 cups coconut oil
- 16 ounces jarred pickle juice
- 2 eggs, whisked

Directions:

1. In a bowl, mix chicken breast pieces with pickle juice, stir, cover and keep in the fridge for 24 hours.
2. Put eggs in a bowl and pork rinds in another one.
3. Dip chicken pieces in egg and then in rings and coat well.

4. Heat up a pan with the oil over medium high heat, add chicken pieces, fry them for 3 minutes on each side, transfer them to paper towels and drain grease.

5. Serve with a keto aioli sauce on the side.

Enjoy!

Nutrition: calories 260, fat 5, fiber 1, carbs 2, protein 20

Chicken Calzone

This special calzone is so delicious!

Preparation time: 10 minutes

Cooking time: 1 hour

Servings: 12

Ingredients:

- 2 eggs
- 1 keto pizza crust
- ½ cup parmesan, grated
- 1 pound chicken breasts, skinless, boneless and each sliced in halves
- ½ cup keto marinara sauce
- 1 teaspoon Italian seasoning
- 1 teaspoon onion powder
- 1 teaspoon garlic powder
- Salt and black pepper to the taste
- ¼ cup flaxseed, ground
- 8 ounces provolone cheese

Directions:

1. In a bowl, mix Italian seasoning with onion powder, garlic powder, salt, pepper, flaxseed and parmesan and stir well.
2. In another bowl, mix eggs with a pinch of salt and pepper and whisk well.
3. Dip chicken pieces in eggs and then in seasoning mix, place all pieces on a lined baking sheet and bake in the oven at 350 degrees F for 30 minutes.
4. Put pizza crust dough on a lined baking sheet and spread half of the provolone cheese on half
5. Take chicken out of the oven, chop and spread over provolone cheese.
6. Add marinara sauce and then the rest of the cheese.
7. Cover all these with the other half of the dough and shape your calzone.
8. Seal its edges, introduce in the oven at 350 degrees F and bake for 20 minutes more.
9. Leave calzone to cool down before slicing and serving.

Enjoy!

Nutrition: calories 340, fat 8, fiber 2, carbs 6, protein 20

Mexican Chicken Soup

It's very simple to make a tasty keto chicken soup! Try this one!

Preparation time: 10 minutes

Cooking time: 4 hours

Servings: 6

Ingredients:

- 1 and ½ pounds chicken tights, skinless, boneless and cubed
- 15 ounces chicken stock
- 15 ounces canned chunky salsa
- 8 ounces Monterey jack

Directions:

1. In your slow cooker, mix chicken with stock, salsa and cheese, stir, cover and cook on High for 4 hours.
2. Uncover pot, stir soup, divide into bowls and serve.

Enjoy!

Nutrition: calories 400, fat 22, fiber 3, carbs 6, protein 38

Simple Chicken Stir Fry

It's a keto friendly recipe you should really try soon!

Preparation time: 10 minutes

Cooking time: 12 minutes

Servings: 2

Ingredients:

- 2 chicken thighs, skinless, boneless cut into thin strips
- 1 tablespoon sesame oil
- 1 teaspoon red pepper flakes
- 1 teaspoon onion powder
- 1 tablespoon ginger, grated
- ¼ cup tamari sauce
- ½ teaspoon garlic powder
- ½ cup water
- 1 tablespoon stevia
- ½ teaspoon xanthan gum
- ½ cup scallions, chopped
- 2 cups broccoli florets

Directions:

1. Heat up a pan with the oil over medium high heat, add chicken and ginger, stir and cook for 3 minutes.
2. Add water, tamari sauce, onion powder, garlic powder, stevia, pepper flakes and xanthan gum, stir and cook for 5 minutes.
3. Add broccoli and scallions, stir, cook for 2 minutes more and divide between plates.
4. Serve hot.

Enjoy!

Nutrition: calories 210, fat 10, fiber 3, carbs 5, protein 20

Spinach And Artichoke Chicken

The combination is really exceptional!

Preparation time: 10 minutes

Cooking time: 50 minutes

Servings: 4

Ingredients:

- 4 ounces cream cheese
- 4 chicken breasts
- 10 ounces canned artichoke hearts, chopped
- 10 ounces spinach
- ½ cup parmesan, grated
- 1 tablespoon dried onion
- 1 tablespoon garlic, dried
- Salt and black pepper to the taste
- 4 ounces mozzarella, shredded

Directions:

1. Place chicken breasts on a lined baking sheet, season with salt and pepper, introduce in the oven at 400 degrees F and bake for 30 minutes.

2. In a bowl, mix artichokes with onion, cream cheese, parmesan, spinach, garlic, salt and pepper and stir.
3. Take chicken out of the oven, cut each piece in the middle, divide artichokes mix, sprinkle mozzarella, introduce in the oven at 400 degrees F and bake for 15 minutes more.
4. Serve hot.

Enjoy!

Nutrition: calories 450, fat 23, fiber 1, carbs 3, protein 39

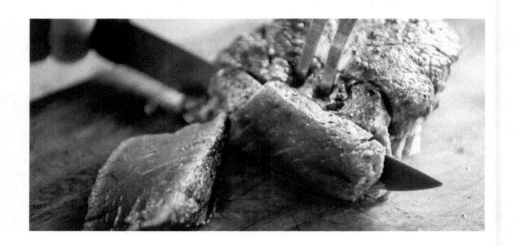

Lightning Source UK Ltd.
Milton Keynes UK
UKHW020214080521
383350UK00003B/277